T0144421

BASIC HEALTH PUBLICATIONS USER'S GUIDE

TO GOOD FATS AND BAD FATS

Learn the Difference Between Fats That Make You Well and Fats That Make You Sick.

MARIE MONEYSMITH

JACK CHALLEM Series Editor

The information contained in this book is based upon the research and personal and professional experiences of the author. It is not intended as a substitute for consulting with your physician or other healthcare provider. Any attempt to diagnose and treat an illness should be done under the direction of a healthcare professional.

The publisher does not advocate the use of any particular healthcare protocol but believes the information in this book should be available to the public. The publisher and author are not responsible for any adverse effects or consequences resulting from the use of the suggestions, preparations, or procedures discussed in this book. Should the reader have any questions concerning the appropriateness of any procedures or preparations mentioned, the author and the publisher strongly suggest consulting a professional healthcare advisor.

Series Editor: Jack Challem
Editor: Rowan Jacobson
Typesetter: Gary A. Rosenberg
Series Cover Designer: Mike Stromberg

Basic Health Publications, Inc.

ISBN: 978-1-59120-052-9 (Pbk.)
ISBN: 978-1-68162-856-1 (Hardcover)

CONTENTS

INTRODUCTION

If you're confused about fat, you've come to the right place. In recent years, experts have taken us from an "all fat is bad" position to the more realistic "some fats are good" stance of today. The problem is that the transition left a lot of confusion in its wake. How can olive oil be healthier than vegetable oil when they seem so much alike? Which is healthier—margarine or butter? What makes one fat good and another bad? How can anyone without an advanced degree in chemistry make sense of it all?

The truth is, sorting out the good fats from the bad is easier than it might seem. And yes, it is worth the effort. Scientists are discovering that getting enough of the good fats—and cutting back on the not-so-good—is crucial to our health in a number of ways. Many experts suspect that some of today's most common diseases could be controlled, or even avoided, with proper fat intake.

Research has shown that good fats can affect a wide range of health conditions, including heart disease, certain types of cancer, high blood pressure, inflammation, type 2 diabetes, rheumatoid and osteoarthritis, kidney disease, digestive disorders (such as ulcerative colitis and Crohn's disease), asthma, emotional disturbances, mental functions, and—last, but far from least—obesity and weight management.

That's right! As strange as it sounds, proper fat intake could help the millions of Americans, 60 percent of the population, who are considered overweight or obese. Why? Because good fats are now considered a key element in weight loss and management.

Maintaining a healthy weight has nothing to do with vanity. Excess pounds set the stage for the serious health conditions mentioned above, and can compromise our health in many other ways. In fact, our ever expanding girth is now considered the second-most common preventable cause of death in this country, after smoking.

Experts cite several reasons for the wave of obesity sweeping the country. One of the most ironic reasons is the explosion in "fat-free" and "low-fat" foods that have flooded supermarket shelves in recent years. These so-called "healthy" foods ballooned into a multibillion-dollar enterprise—at the same time that more and more Americans were growing heavier, and failing to get healthier! Clearly, something is wrong with this picture.

Part of the problem was that consumers were lured into the false belief that anything with less fat was good for their health and would help with weight loss. In fact, just the opposite was true. To replace the flavor lost by the lack of fat (fat carries flavor), most of these foods are loaded with sugar, which is a simple carbohydrate and packs plenty of calories—but virtually no nutrition. Is it any surprise people could eat less fat and still put on pounds?

Meanwhile, the other health benefits associated with low-fat diets failed to materialize, too. Heart disease, cancer, and stroke are still the leading causes of death in the United States, according to the Centers for Disease Control. In 1999 the numbers of deaths were just about the same for all three conditions as they were in 1981. Clearly, the low-fat plan did not lower the risk of developing the most common diseases.

The second part of the problem involves the confusion about fat. First, we were told to eliminate fat from our diets, period. Then word started getting out that some fats were okay, but others weren't. Meanwhile, the diet gurus were arguing over which eating plan was best (High protein? High carbs? No carbs?). No wonder weary consumers threw their hands up in the air and simply gave up.

Obviously, the notion that fat is the enemy is an oversimplification. The truth is, we need fat. Or, more accurately, we need the right types of fat. With those, our brains and nervous systems function better, we absorb vitamins properly, our hair and skin look and feel more attractive, and our cardiovascular and immune systems work as they should.

Of course, all fat is not created equal. Just as there are advantages to consuming good fats, there are disadvantages to getting too many bad fats. Unfortunately, the typical American diet provides us with far too much of the bad variety in snack, processed, fried, and fast foods. And, to add insult to injury, diligent consumers who read food labels may think what they're eating is better than it really is. Why? Because nutrition labels don't list the worst offenders in the fat family.

In between the health-friendly fats and those that damage our health, there are other assorted fats with both upsides and downsides. Some provide relief for specific conditions; others have surprised researchers with their recently discovered health benefits. Yet with some experts telling us we are eating too much fat, and others insisting we aren't getting enough of the right ones, no wonder confusion reigns. Sorting out the good fats from the bad is what this book is all about, and yes, it can be done. We need to rethink fat, get to know the players, and start using more good fats in our diet to improve our health, not diminish it.

CHAPTER 1

FATS: THE GOOD, THE BAD, AND THE HEALTHY

In a perfect world, there would be no conflicting studies, contradictory experts, or confusion over something as simple as fat. Our world is not there yet, but that's no excuse for letting the lack of straight answers prevent you from staying healthy.

First, let's set the record straight: fat is not the enemy. In fact, in many ways, fat is our friend. It cushions many of our internal organs and provides insulation that protects us against plummeting temperatures—something our Ice Age ancestors probably appreciated much more than we do.

Fat is one of three macro-nutrients in our diets, along with protein and carbohydrates. All food calories are made up of these three types of molecules. But fat is by far the richest energy source in our diets. Protein and carbohydrates both contain about 60 calories per tablespoonful, while fat contains more than twice this much—approximately 135 per tablespoonful, making it an excellent source of energy, but clearly one that should be used in moderation. Most of us could survive

Men, Women, and Fat

Men store less body fat—roughly 16 percent of their weight—than women, who typically store about 25 percent of their body weight as fat.

for thirty or forty days with water alone if necessary, simply by using our fat reserves.

On average, about 34 percent of our daily calories come from fat or oil, which is simply a liquid form of fat. Considering that the American Heart Association, the National Cancer Institute, and many other health organizations and experts recommend keeping that figure at about 30 percent, the 4 percent difference seems trivial. In fact, it looks as though we are doing pretty well at taming our taste for fat. But unfortunately, that's not quite true, as the growing number of Americans with a weight problem shows.

Fat Sources
When we consume more carbohydrates than we use in daily activities, these get stored as body fat, just as dietary fat does.

What's so bad about carrying around a few extra pounds? More than you think. Researchers at Brigham and Women's Hospital and Harvard Medical School examined more than 120,000 middle-aged people and found that heavier folk were at a greater risk of developing heart disease, high blood pressure, type 2 diabetes, stroke, colon cancer, and gallstones than thinner individuals. The highest number of health problems occurred in those most overweight. But even a few extra pounds increased the likelihood of developing at least one chronic health condition.

Extra Weight Endangers Health

Although we have a national obsession with weight, the Centers for Disease Control (CDC) statistics show that cardiovascular disease remains the nation's leading cause of death (more than 700,000 annually), followed by cancer (about 550,000) and stroke (166,000). Fat plays a role in all three. Good fats can protect us from developing these illnesses, and in many cases can ease symptoms, while bad fats are risk factors for all three leading causes of death.

Of course, the number of deaths doesn't tell the whole story. Millions of individuals continue to live in the shadow of cardiovascular disease, cancer, or complications from a past stroke, while millions of others suffer from diabetes, arthritis, and depression. Here again, fat plays an important part in the development of these conditions and their impact on our lives.

Take cardiovascular disease (CVD), for example. This is really an umbrella term, comprised of heart disease (also known as coronary artery disease), stroke, high blood pressure, and congestive heart failure. The American Heart Association reports that some 62 million Americans have been diagnosed with at least one element of cardiovascular disease, and many of them suffer from two or more, such as heart disease and high blood pressure.

Women and Heart Disease

Although women tend to be more concerned about breast cancer, they are ten times more likely to die of CVD than breast cancer.

One of the most familiar elements of cardiovascular disease is atherosclerosis, or hardening of the arteries. This occurs when arteries become clogged with deposits of plaque: small clumps formed when the waxlike fat known as cholesterol combines with other substances in the blood. As the plaque continues to accumulate, blood flow through the artery is slowed. When this occurs in the artery that supplies the heart with blood, it is known as coronary artery disease. Like rocks or logs in a river, these impediments gather clusters of blood cells, creating a larger blockage, and eventually blood cannot pass through the artery at all. Deprived of oxygen, the heart sends signals in the form of chest or arm pain, and finally a heart attack.

During the past few decades, experts have advised us that the best way to avoid a heart attack, or stroke—which is simply a blocked artery to the brain instead of the heart—is to lower our fat intake and reduce cholesterol levels. In theory, with less fat and cholesterol in the bloodstream, there is less likelihood of an artery becoming blocked.

Many people who had been diagnosed with high levels of cholesterol cut back on the most notorious cholesterol-producing foods—red meat, eggs, and full-fat dairy products. An entire industry sprang up around low-fat and fat-free fare. Still, the overall number of heart attacks remained fairly steady.

Why? Experts are discovering that simply keeping fat out of the diet was too simplistic. For example, researchers at the Harvard School of Public Health have noted two things. First, it's clear that *the type of fat*, not the total amount of fat, is what correlates to cholesterol levels. And second, increasing the amount of good fats, known as *omega-3s*, and maintaining a balance between these and a group known as *omega-6s*, are the keys to lowering risk of heart attack.

Low Fat Leads to More Pounds

Meanwhile, the focus on eliminating fat from the diet created an unexpected new problem—weight gain. According to the CDC, the number of obese Americans has nearly doubled in the past two decades. Today, more than half—61 percent, to be precise—of the adult population in this country is either overweight or obese, a condition that costs us $117 billion a year in increased health care costs.

Health experts use the body mass index (BMI) to determine who is overweight and who is obese. (Check your own BMI at the National Heart, Lung, and Blood Institute's website: nhlbisupport.com/bmi/bmicalc.htm) A BMI between 25 and 29.9 is defined as overweight. Anyone with a BMI of 30 or above is considered obese.

How did cutting back on fat make us fat? In the rush to avoid fat, we filled our shopping carts with low-fat versions of cookies, doughnuts, chips, and frozen meals, without noticing that these "good" choices often had as many—if not more—calories than the regular versions. In essence, we simply traded fat for carbohydrates, and ate more because we mistakenly believed "low fat" was a license to indulge.

Fat Definitions
Legally, the term "fat free" means less than 0.5 grams of fat in one serving. "Low fat" is defined as 3 grams or less in a serving.

A Fat Primer

To make smart choices about fat, you first need to know some basic information. Let's start with those familiar terms found on food labels: "monounsaturated," "polyunsaturated," and "saturated." These terms classify fats by the number of hydrogen atoms that are paired with carbon atoms in the fat molecules. A monounsaturated fat has one double bond between carbon atoms to make up for missing hydrogen. The one double bond makes it "mono," from the Greek word for "one." A fat that is missing more than one hydrogen atom and has multiple bonds between carbon atoms is called polyunsaturated, "poly" meaning "many." When all the carbon atoms in a fat molecule have hydrogen partners, the fat is considered "saturated," or completely filled.

A less technical way to recognize a saturated fat is the solid form it takes at room temperature. Butter, shortening, lard, and the marbling in meat are saturated fats. Conversely, both monounsaturated fats (olive and canola oils, for example) and polyunsaturated fats (corn, safflower, and most other vegetable oils) are liquid at room temperature.

Confused? Here's a bit of help. A good mnemonic device for keeping track of which fats are good and bad is to remember that their alphabetical order is also a listing of their health order. Monounsaturated fats are best, followed by polyunsaturated, and finally the "only in small amounts" saturated fat.

Although we tend to think that foods contain only one type of fat, the truth is a little different. All three fatty acids are present in most foods. Olive oil, for example, widely considered to be a monounsaturated fat, also contains small amounts of polyunsaturated and saturated fats. And salmon, a good source of healthy monounsaturated fats, contains a little saturated fat as well. For simplicity's sake, the dominant fat (that is, the fat most common in the food) determines the category the food falls in.

A Few Words about Bad Fats

As you are probably aware, saturated fat, found primarily in meat and dairy products, is not one of the good fats. Saturated fat's bad reputation comes from its tendency to raise levels of "bad" LDL (low-density lipoprotein) cholesterol and lower the "good" HDL (high-density lipoprotein) variety. But it does have one advantage: because all its carbon atoms are connected to hydrogen atoms, it is more stable than unsaturated fats. That means it stays fresh longer, and doesn't go rancid as quickly as the unsaturated oils. Unfortunately, that doesn't make it good for you. In Chapter 6, we'll look at this bad fat in more depth.

Cholesterol

HDL ("good") cholesterol cleanses our arteries, keeps cell structure intact, and produces hormones, while LDL ("bad") cholesterol increases risk of heart disease, stroke, and other diseases.

You have probably heard the term "partially hydrogenated vegetable oil." In this process, hydrogen and heat are added to a polyunsaturated oil to make it a solid, like margarine. The goal is to make the oil more stable, and less likely to turn bad. Although this seems fairly innocent, fats known as trans-saturated fatty acids, or just trans fats, which damage hearts and arteries, are created during the process. As a result, partially hydrogenated oils should be avoided.

Meet the Most Famous Fat of All

There is one other member of the fat family you are no doubt familiar with—cholesterol. While the common wisdom about cholesterol is that it should be avoided, it's important to know that experts do not consider this fat to be as harmful as trans fats or saturated fat. Here's why: cholesterol is actually produced in our bodies, and it performs a long list of beneficial functions. In fact, it's vital to our health and well being. It's used in hormone production, maintenance of cell membrane flexibility, and digestion of fats. Cholesterol also helps keep our skin healthy and is a source of vitamin D, a necessity for calcium absorption.

Cholesterol's bad reputation stems from the problems that can occur when it accumulates in the arteries. If blood flow through the arteries is restricted by a buildup of cholesterol-based plaque, the result can be a stroke, heart attack, or other serious conditions. In addition, researchers are now discovering there may be a link between high cholesterol and Alzheimer's, the increasingly common brain-damaging disease.

Blood Test Terms

Triglycerides are fats circulating in the bloodstream. Lipoproteins are combinations of fat and protein that transport fats in the bloodstream.

The cholesterol in food comes in only one form. But if you've ever had a blood panel done during a visit to the doctor, you know that there are different types of cholesterol in our bodies. Experts now subdivide cholesterol into several different categories, in - cluding "good" HDL and "bad" LDL.

Our bodies need both LDL and HDL cholesterol, but in the right proportions. Ideally, total cholesterol should be less than 200 mg per dL (deciliter). Total cholesterol levels of more than 240 mg/dL are considered a risk factor for heart disease. But the cholesterol totals are less important than the ratio of HDL to LDL. It's best to keep the bad, LDL cholesterol levels below 100. Anything above 100 increases heart disease risk, especially levels that top 130. These figures apply to both men and women. HDL cholesterol levels for men should be 40 mg/dL or more, while women's levels should be in the 50–60 range.

Unfortunately, the typical American diet provides us with far more LDL cholesterol than we need, along with too little HDL. And it is this imbalance that tips the scales toward heart problems and other health conditions. Snacks, processed foods, and fast foods tend to be loaded with the worst forms of fat: saturated and trans. Many of these products are labeled "cholesterol free," which is technically true. But all our bodies need is a heaping portion of the bad fats to go on a cholesterol-producing spree. Not only that, the cholesterol being produced tends to be of the bad LDL variety. To make matters worse, HDL cholesterol levels drop on a diet high in saturated fats. In addition, too much saturated and trans fats can prevent our bodies from fully utilizing the good fats they do get.

Speaking of good fats, what happens to our cholesterol when we consume the good instead of the bad? As you might expect, the results are very different. In most cases, a meal rich in the beneficial monounsaturated fats can help lower LDL cholesterol without reducing HDL levels.

Polyunsaturated vegetable oils (such as corn, safflower, soy, sesame, and sunflower) are less healthy than the monounsaturated variety. While they can lower LDL cholesterol, HDL levels tend to drop, too. Polyunsaturated fats are some of the most common fats in our diet. If you look through your pantry or refrigerator, you're very likely to find at least one of these in a sauce, salad dressing, or snack food. These fats are not dietary disasters, like saturated and trans fats. The body relies on them to create substances that help regulate inflammation, and our cells put polyunsaturated fats to work shoring up membranes to protect the cell's contents. Because of this, for years we've been told to choose these vegetable oils, and the food industry often advertises products as being "made with pure safflower oil" or a similar, seemingly healthy fat. But the truth is these all-too-common polyunsaturated vegetable oils take a backseat to monounsaturated fats when it comes to health benefits.

Ideally, olive oil and other monounsaturated fats should comprise 10 to 15 percent of your total daily calories, while polyunsaturated fats should account for only 5 to 10 percent.

Close-Up on Monounsaturated Fats

Monounsaturated fats are made up of monounsaturated fatty acids, the heroes of the fat world. These heart-healthy compounds have the unique ability to lower bad LDL cholesterol levels without changing the HDL levels. They also transport vitamins and other healthy substances, lower blood pressure, and protect against certain diseases, like diabetes. In addition, monounsaturated fats fight inflammation, which is now being recognized as a factor in everything from arthritis to heart disease.

Spoiled Oils
Unsaturated fats can turn rancid quickly if not refrigerated. Rancid oil contains harmful free radicals, smells like oil paint, and should be thrown out.

Monounsaturated fats are plentiful in olive, canola, and peanut oil, as well as almonds, avocados, olives, and pecans. Of all these sources, olive oil has had the most attention, probably because it is the oil of choice in the much-praised "Mediterranean diet," modeled after the eating habits of residents of Greece, Southern Italy, and Spain. People living in this region are known for having a very low incidence of coronary artery disease. Experts attribute this to their diet, a combination of vegetables, grains, fish, and olive oil, the last of which makes up about 30 percent of their daily caloric intake.

Studies have repeatedly shown that olive oil is truly a good fat. A *Nutrition Review* summary of previously published research noted that olive oil's health benefits may include "reduction of risk factors of coronary heart disease, prevention of several varieties of cancers, and modification of immune and inflammatory responses." That's an impressive list of benefits, especially considering that we are not talking about a prescription drug or new medicine, but a delicious part of the everyday diet.

Now that you have a solid foundation in the basics of good fat, let's take a look at a different piece of the puzzle—the essential fatty acids (EFAs).

More Good News—The Essential Fatty Acids

You may have heard the term *essential fatty acids*, or the abbreviation *EFAs*. These are a special class of fats, and, as their name implies, the EFAs are absolutely essential for good health. EFAs can't be produced by our bodies, so they must be obtained from foods or supplements. During the no-fat frenzy of recent years, we threw out the baby with the bathwater by avoiding these vital nutrients. Today, experts are recommending the EFAs for a variety of conditions, including everything from heart health to treating ADHD.

There are three different categories of EFAs: omega-3s, also known as alpha-linoleic acid (ALA); omega-6s, or linolenic acid (LA); and omega-9s (oleic acid). Don't be intimidated by these terms; read on and you'll quickly become accustomed to them. The one you really want to pay attention to is *omega-3*. This is not because the omega-6s and omega-9s are harmful per se, but because the omega-3s are the ones most lacking in our diets. The EFAs are not listed on food labels yet, but with a little learning you will know where to find them.

Essential Fatty Acids
Substances found in fat that are vital to good health, but which our bodies cannot make. We must get them from food or supplements.

The EFAs are classified as polyunsaturated fats. There is a long list of health benefits bestowed on us by EFAs, many of them similar to those provided by monounsaturated and polyunsaturated fats. They are involved, for example, in everything from creating new cells and repairing old ones to mental and nervous system functions, as well as emotional and heart health. The key to getting the most from EFAs is a properly balanced intake of omega-3s and omega-6s. (Another type of fatty acid, known as the omega-9s, is also vital for good health, but, unlike the omega-3s and 6s, our bodies can manufacture omega-9s.) In the next chapters, we'll look at these fatty acids and see why experts think many of today's most common illnesses are a result of an EFA imbalance in our diet.

CHAPTER 2

OMEGA-3
FATTY ACIDS

Difficulty learning, erratic behavior, weakness, coordination problems—these are only a few of the problems caused by a lack of omega-3 fatty acids. Could some people actually be deficient in our well-fed nation? Absolutely, say authorities. A diet overly rich in omega-6 fatty acids, which are plentiful in our daily fare, can tip the balance and create an omega-3 shortfall.

Before looking at how that happens, let's get an overview of the omega-3 family and its benefits. Omega-3s are found in far fewer foods than are omega-6s. Back in the days when livestock grazed in fields and chickens scratched for food in barnyards, meat and eggs were decent sources of omega-3s, simply because the animals ate plants with high omega-3 content. By contrast, today's meat and eggs are filled with omega-6s from the grains animals are fed. (If you're willing to do a little legwork, you can still find grass-fed beef and eggs laid by chickens fed flaxseeds and other omega-3 rich foods. These products contain higher levels of omega-3s than factory-farmed foods. Ask in your local health-food store or coop.)

Omega-3s come in three types: alpha-linolenic acid (ALA), docosahexaenoic acid (DHA), and eicosapentaenoic acid (EPA). DHA and EPA are abundant in fatty fish, such as salmon, sardines, mackerel, anchovies, halibut, tuna, and sea bass. The best source of ALA is flax, both the seeds and the oil derived from them. Other good sources of ALA are dark, leafy greens, canola oil, hempseeds, walnuts, wheat germ, and soybeans, as well as the oils from these plants. Purslane, which is considered a weed in this country, is an ALA-rich plant that is widely used in cooking in the rest of the world.

The benefits of all the omega-3s are impressive and occur throughout the body, including the cardiovascular system, glucose management, bones, and even brain health. Some of the best evidence of omega-3's heart-saving abilities, for example, comes from the follow-up to the four-year Lyon Diet Heart Study, which examined the Mediterranean diet's ability to protect against a second heart attack. The Mediterranean diet relies heavily on fish, fruits, vegetables, and grains, as well as healthy oils. (This particular study used canola oil, although olive oil is a traditional staple of the Mediterranean diet.) Researchers concluded that eating a typical Mediterranean diet was responsible for reducing the risk of second heart attacks among the study's 600 participants by as much as 70 percent! Other similar studies have confirmed that an ALA-rich diet reduces death from heart attacks and other causes.

But our hearts aren't the only thing that benefits from ALA. When participants in a study at the University of Toronto were fed up to 50 grams daily of ALA-rich ground flaxseeds, they had a nearly 30 percent de - crease in blood sugar levels after meals. This is an im- portant benefit for anyone concerned about developing insulin resistance or the con- dition known as syndrome X.

Syndrome X
A cluster of health problems including insulin resistance, high cholesterol and triglycerides, excess weight, and high blood pressure.

Omega-3s can make bones stronger in postmenopausal women, too, by decreasing the body's produc- tion of inflammatory, bone-damaging proteins called cytokines. A study published in *Alter - native Medicine Review* noted that supple- ments of fish oil, flaxseeds, and flaxseed oil all provided this benefit, while simultaneously increasing calcium absorption, bone density, and bone calcium.

Last, but not least, an animal study in Australia produced intriguing results, showing that a diet rich in omega-3s was much more effective than a low-fat diet when it came to fighting the negative effects caused by previ- ous consumption of large amounts of saturated fats. So diets high in omega-3 fats may protect against obesity.

Fish Oil for Health

During the low-fat craze, researchers were at a loss to explain an anomaly. How could Green - land's native populations and North America's Inuits live on a nearly all-fat diet and still have remarkably low rates of heart disease? The explanation turned out to be the omega-3 con- tent of the fish and marine animals they were eating.

Since then, the fish oils known as DHA and EPA have been extensively studied in relation to health. The overall results are outstanding. Fish oils provide protection against a wide range of conditions involving our cardiovascular, emotional, immune, and neurological systems. Inflammatory conditions like rheumatoid arthritis and osteoarthritis, asthma, multiple sclerosis, breast cancer, schizophrenia, depression, bipolar disorder, and a host of other common ailments all respond to treatment with fish oil. These omega-3s also fight hardening of the arteries and can lower triglyceride levels in the blood, while helping reduce the "stickiness" that makes blood platelets clump together. Fish oils have also shown promise in regulating dangerous heart arrhythmias.

Platelets
Small, disk-shaped bodies in the blood that promote clotting, but, when clumped in hardened arteries, can cause heart attacks and strokes.

A sampling of recent studies shows just how effective the omega-3 fish oils can be. As you probably know, more Americans die of heart disease each year than of any other cause, but two recent clinical trials confirm that fish is heart-healthy for both men and women. The first study, reported in the respected *New England Journal of Medicine,* involved 22,000 men, and found that those who had the highest blood levels of omega-3 fatty acids were 90 percent less likely to die suddenly from a heart attack. The second study appeared in the highly regarded *Journal of the American Medical Association* and involved nearly 90,000 women. This time, researchers found that women who ate the most fish and omega-3 fatty acids had a lower risk of both heart disease and death from heart attacks.

Exactly how fish oil protects us from heart

disease isn't yet known, but one theory involves omega-3's ability to keep our blood vessels flexible, thereby preventing the dangerous blood clots that cause heart attacks and strokes. Heart experts, who now believe hardening of the arteries plays a greater role in heart disease than was previously thought, are searching for ways to keep arteries flexible, and it seems that fish oil may be the solution.

A randomized, placebo-controlled, double-blind study tested the ability of EPA and DHA to ward off hardening of the arteries, a factor that causes both high blood pressure and heart attacks. There was a 36 percent increase in arterial flexibility among patients taking EPA, and a 27 percent increase for those receiving DHA, but the placebo group did not experience any significant benefits.

Fish Oil Helps More Than the Heart

As mentioned earlier, fish oil is effective for treating a wide range of conditions. One of these is insulin resis - tance, a precursor to type 2 diabetes and syndrome X. Research presented during the Annual Experimental Biology 2002 Conference suggests that the fish oil DHA can improve insulin resistance. After just three months of DHA supplements (1.8 grams every morning), 70 percent of the study participants, all of whom began the study with insulin resistance, had improved insulin function, and the change was clinically significant for fully 50 percent of them.

The Diabetes Epidemic

The number of people with type 2, or adult-onset, diabetes is increasing at an epidemic rate. Millions of people who have the disease are not aware of it.

A growing body of research also shows that multiple sclerosis (MS) patients improve after taking fish oil. In Norway, researchers found that a combination of fish oil capsules, vitamin supplementation, and dietary advice improved symptoms in a group of newly diagnosed MS patients. Experts noted that blood levels of omega-3s rose during the two years of the study, while levels of omega-6s decreased significantly, which suggests that correcting the balance of omega-3s was one reason why fish oil helped.

The benefits of fish oil extend to our brains, too. You may have heard people claim "fish is brain food." Recent studies with DHA confirm this belief. The importance of this substance to healthy brains begins in the womb: a clearly established link exists between sufficient supplies of omega-3s, especially DHA, and the development of a fetus's nervous system. In infancy, babies also need ample amounts of DHA for healthy growth and development. Vision, brain functions, and the nervous system all appear to benefit from this omega-3. These health advantages help explain why DHA is abundant in breast milk.

Food for Thought
Our brains are 50–60 percent fat, with high levels of omega-3s, which explains why this nutrient enhances brain functions and eases emotional difficulties.

Even after infancy, fish oils can help keep children healthy. DHA deficiencies are associated with ADHD, depression, cystic fibrosis, and hostile aggression. Fish oils can also help ease children's asthma symptoms. A randomized, placebo-controlled study found that children given daily doses of fish oil supplements—a combination of DHA and EPA—had reduced bronchial asthma symptoms and experienced no significant side effects. Meanwhile, there were no benefits among children in the control group.

What about vegetarians, who don't find fish oil supplements any more appealing than fish itself, or vegans, who don't eat eggs? Good news! There is a fish-free way to get the omega-3 health benefits—the tiny seeds of the flax plant.

Make Friends with Flax

Fish oil may have had more media attention than flaxseeds, but it would be a mistake to overlook the benefits of flax. Best known as the raw material from which linen is made, the hardy flax plant has been treasured for its medicinal abilities for centuries. In the Middle East, for example, ancient cultures used the seeds to ease digestive and respiratory problems. Today, they are becoming an increasingly popular addition to the daily diet, in both food and supplement form.

Many experts believe flaxseeds and flax-seed oil can be used as a substitute for fish oil, because the ALA in flax is considered the "mother" EFA. With sufficient supplies of ALA, a healthy person's body should be able to produce DHA and EPA. There is some controversy, however, about how effectively the body does this, especially as we age.

Research has shown that flax can reduce problems associated with cardiovascular disease, as well as certain cancers. Flaxseed oil helps lower blood pressure, bad LDL cholesterol levels, and triglycerides, while keeping arteries flexible and preventing blood platelets from clumping together to create life-threat-ening blood clots. Flaxseeds also fight breast cancer by slowing tumor growth and making breast tissue less vulnerable to cancer cells. Recently, French scientists discovered further proof of the link between flaxseeds and breast health when they found that women with the highest levels of ALA in their breast tissues were least likely to develop cancer. No other EFA provided this protection.

Flax for Arthritis
Studies have shown that flaxseed oil safely and effectively relieves the pain and inflammation of osteoarthritis.

Oil versus Seeds

Although flaxseeds and flaxseed oil have a lot in common, they appear to have slightly different health benefits. For example, the seeds contain lignans, which provide protection against certain toxins. Fortunately, there are flaxseed oils available that contain lignans. Or you can hedge your bets and use both oil and seeds. The nut-like flavor of flaxseeds is a tasty addition to cereals, stews, soups, or yogurt. Be advised, though, that the seeds must be ground into small pieces to be digested and release their health benefits. A small coffee grinder does a good job of this.

Lignans
Plant fibers that fight cancer-causing substances and help prevent tumors from forming.

Perilla Oil: The New Kid on the Block

So far, most of the fats and oils we've looked at have been fairly commonplace. But there is one exotic-sounding oil you should know about, since it is likely to become increasingly popular, and that is perilla oil. A favorite in Asia, where it has been a cooking staple for centuries, perilla oil is derived from the ruffle-edged leaves of the perilla plant, a dark, leafy vegetable available in red and green varieties. Perilla oil can be found in this country now, although you may have to do some detective work to locate it. If you can't find perilla oil at your health food store, check out Asian markets in your area.

Perilla oil has not been as extensively studied as fish and flaxseed oils, but the research that has been done shows that this ALA-rich oil can accomplish many of the same feats as the other omega-3 sources, including: protecting the heart by reducing the "stickiness" of blood platelets, decreasing the likelihood of life-threatening blood clots; enhancing the immune system; fighting pain and inflammation; and alleviating asthma and allergic reactions, while improving lung functions. An animal study reported that perilla oil inhibits the growth of tumors of the breast, colon, and kidney more effectively than do safflower or soybean oil.

Perilla oil has other benefits as well. As noted earlier, when our bodies have access to ALA, we should be able to process our own DHA and EPA, but we have greater difficulty making the conversion as we age. A recent study, however, found that when elderly subjects were given three grams of perilla oil daily for ten months, blood levels of EPA and DHA increased substantially without any negative side effects.

Since there are so few studies with perilla oil and human subjects, it is difficult to determine the effects of long-term supplementation. We do know, however, that perilla oil is commonly used in Asian cuisine and has not been linked to any negative side effects. And there is one other advantage: perilla oil is far less expensive than some other forms of omega-3s.

CHAPTER 3

BALANCING ACT: OMEGA-6 FATTY ACIDS

Like the omega-3 fatty acids, the omega-6s are also important to overall good health, especially when it comes to development and normal growth. The omega-6s fall into two categories: linoleic acid (LA), and gamma linolenic acid (GLA), plus a close cousin named conjugated linoleic acid (CLA). The richest sources of the omega-6s are the familiar safflower, corn, sunflower, sesame, cottonseed, and soy oils, along with the less well-known hempseed, walnut, evening primrose, and borage oils.

There is no doubt that omega-6s are good for us. They are, after all, classified as essential fatty acids. But, unlike the omega-3s, which most of us need to consume in greater amounts, the omega-6s are already far too plentiful in the American diet. Check out the labels of such everyday foods as margarine, salad dressing, chips, crackers, and ready-made baked goods. You'll find safflower, corn, sunflower, or soy oil in all these products.

Obviously, it's very easy to get omega-6s at meal time. But compare the availability of omega-6s in our diets to the scarcity of omega-3s, and you'll see why it can be a challenge to get roughly equal amounts of these important nutrients, as experts prescribe. While the proper ratio of omega-6s to omega-3s is 1:1, the typical American consumes roughly a 20:1 ratio or worse. The bottom line: without balanced intake of omega-3s and omega-6s, our health suffers. We get fewer of the omega-3 benefits to our cardiovascular and nervous systems, and good HDL cholesterol levels may drop, a side effect of too many omega-6s.

Eating Like Our Ancestors

Experts estimate that the ideal ratio of omega-3s to omega-6s is 1:1, an amount similar to what our very earliest ancestors consumed. Remember, our bodies have not evolved all that much since prehistoric times, but our diet has undergone a major revolution. The earliest humans had to work hard for each meal. They chased down game and roamed far and wide in search of berries, nuts, greens, and roots. They ate when they were successful, not on a regular, three-meals-a-day basis. Food was rich in omega-3s, whether it was the greens and seeds they consumed or the animals, fish, and birds raised on grass, algae, and seeds. As a result, our ancestors' intake of omega-3s and omega-6s was about equal.

Today, everything has changed. The tremendous amounts of safflower, sunflower, soy, and corn oils, as well as partially hydrogenated fats in our diet, have skewed the ratio heavily in favor of omega-6s. How does this affect us? In several ways, all crucial to our health. First, as we know, our bodies can convert the "mother" omega-3, ALA, into both DHA and EPA, using enzymes to make the chemical conversion. This process won't work, however, if the body has to deal with an overabundance of saturated fats, sugar, or omega-6s, which monopolize the enzymes needed to convert ALA. In other words, even if you are getting a good supply of omega-3s from food or supplements, they may not be able to do their job if your diet is loaded with the most common ingredients in American supermarkets. It is this scenario that sets the stage for potentially serious health problems. Fortunately, restoring the all-important balance between these nutrients is possible with the right good fats.

How Balanced EFAs Make Us Healthier

A healthy balance between omega-3s and omega-6s is important for controlling inflammation. There are times when inflammation can be a good thing. For instance, if you are sick or injured, inflammation provides extra blood and immune cells that target the condition. The swelling that occurs when you sprain your ankle is a good example. This type of inflammation is part of the healing process. When the damaged tissues in the ankle are repaired, the inflammation goes away. But chronic, long-term inflammation is not healthy. In fact, it is associated with serious health complications, including arthritis.

Inflammation Hurts More Than Joints

Many experts believe that inflammation is involved in cardiovascular disease, too, making it a risk factor for heart attacks.

Omega-3s and omega-6s are the raw materials our bodies use to produce prostaglandins—powerful, hormonelike substances used throughout the body to regulate a wide range of functions, including blood pressure, the gastrointestinal system, blood stickiness, and inflammation. Prostaglandins made from omega-3s tend to reduce inflammation, thin the blood, and discourage cell production, while those that originate from omega-6s do the opposite—increase cell production, stimulate inflammation, and increase blood platelet stickiness and clotting.

If your EFA intake is balanced, then prostaglandins are produced in a balanced ratio, too. But when there are more omega-6–based prostaglandins being created, there is a greater likelihood of developing conditions such as arthritis, heart attacks or strokes, or ailments involving uncontrolled cell growth, like cancer. When inflammation becomes a chronic condition, it is a sign of an imbalance in prostaglandin production, a factor directly related to the imbalance of omega-3s and omega-6s in the body.

Good Fats Are a Good Treatment for Inflammation

Traditional medicine has no cure for inflammation. It treats the symptoms with nonsteroidal, anti-inflammatory drugs (NSAIDs), such as Aleve, Advil, and good old aspirin. NSAIDs prevent pain by blocking production of the enzymes COX-1 and COX-2, generators of the "bad" prostaglandins that let inflammation run amok. Unfor- tunately, NSAIDs also block the formation of "good" prostaglandins, a process that can lead to serious side effects.

Wallet Pain
We spend about $2 billion a year on pain-relieving NSAIDs in the United States, even though these drugs do not cure anything.

Not long ago, researchers came up with what seemed to be a solution. After discovering that COX-1 enzymes actually protect the kidneys and digestive tract, they targeted the more damaging COX-2 enzymes with a new generation of drugs aptly named COX-2 inhibitors. For a time it seemed that the COX-2 inhibitors were able to tame inflammation without the side effects of NSAIDs. But, based on newer studies, it appears the COX-2 group is no safer than its predecessors.

Knowing that prostaglandins made from omega-3s reduce inflammation, while those made from omega-6s do the opposite, it stands to reason that increasing omega-3s and decreasing omega-6s would combat arthritis. And that is exactly what happened when scientists at Cardiff University in Wales used omega-3 fatty acids to treat osteoarthritic cartilage from human subjects. Not only did the omega-3s prevent the formation of substances that cause inflammation in cartilage, but they also decreased the factors that cause the destruction of cartilage.

Inflammation can also be involved in cardiovascular health. And here, too, omega-3s have shown an ability to reduce that risk factor. In a randomized, placebo-controlled, double-blind study of more than 200 people, omega-3s, 6s, and 9s were tested for their ability to reduce substances that cause inflammation in the arteries. Only the group that was given 1.5 grams of omega-3s daily benefited from a reduction in arterial inflammation.

Now that you understand why it's important to aim for roughly equal amounts of omega-3s and 6s, look for ways to avoid the most popular omega-6 oils—the ones found primarily in snacks, prepackaged foods, and fast foods, like corn, cottonseed, safflower, and sunflower. These particular oils come up short in health advantages, and so do the foods they are found in. Replace those oils with omega-3s or omega-6s with documented health benefits, like GLA and CLA.

Getting to Know GLA

GLA, a member of the omega-6 family, can be made by our bodies from linoleic acid (LA). But production is slowed by a variety of factors, including everything from aging to high cho-lesterol to alcohol consumption. It is difficult to get GLA from food. It is found in the oil of only a few plant seeds, including borage, black cur-rant, hemp, and evening primrose. Of these oils, only hemp is particularly pleasing in taste, so GLA is usually consumed as a supplement.

Why supplement your diet with GLA? Be-cause this little-known substance has some impressive health benefits. GLA has been shown to lower cholesterol (both total and LDL levels); to treat diabetic neuropathy, rheuma-toid arthritis and other in-flammatory diseases; and to relieve symptoms of PMS, eczema, and the circulatory disorder known as Raynaud's phenomenon. In the case of PMS, for instance, GLA has been shown to ease breast pain and cramps by reduc-ing the inflammation that occurs when the uterus sheds its lining each month. Typically, GLA-rich evening primrose oil is recommended for PMS, but black currant or borage oils are excellent sources of GLA, too.

Fight PMS with GLA
To be effective against PMS, GLA must be taken on a daily basis for at least one menstrual cycle, as it takes up to two months to reach full effectiveness.

Although GLA is widely popular for treating PMS, it is actually shaping up as a true star among good fats. Recent research indicates, for example, that GLA is a powerful anticancer agent. Brazilian researchers tested GLA's ability to fight tumors in animals and found it could "greatly decrease" tumor size, while an injected combination of substances, including GLA and the fish oil EPA, caused a type of brain tumor to go into regression without damaging surrounding tissues. A similar combination of omega-3s and omega-6s also prevented animals from developing chemically induced diabetes.

There are two more benefits to add to this already impressive list. Recent studies show that GLA provides cardiovascular and kidney protection for the elderly, and, in an animal trial, it also decreased the amount of body fat mass compared to a diet based on safflower oil.

CLA Comes to the Fore

Years ago, cows grazed in grassy pastures for much of the year. As a result, whole milk, butter, and beef, all regular features on the American dinner table, were filled with a nutrient called conjugated linoleic acid (CLA), which the cows manufactured from the grass they ate. Ironically, no one knew CLA, a close chemical cousin to linoleic acid (LA), existed until the 1980s, and by then most cattle were fed a grain diet, so they produced very little CLA. Researchers who have studied the health benefits of CLA believe this shortage could be behind the high number of cancer deaths, obesity, and other serious health conditions, including hardening of the arteries, allergies, asthma, and diabetes.

When it comes to improving clogged arteries, CLA has produced outstanding results, such as those obtained during a recent study at the University of Pennsylvania. Researchers were so astonished to find a 30 percent reduction in arterial plaque among animals fed CLA that they repeated the experiment to verify their results. Sure enough, the second study also showed a 30 percent reduction.

Moreover, CLA appears to be an impressive weapon in the war on cancer, especially of the breast, skin, stomach, and colon. High levels of CLA in body tissues are known to be associated with a reduced risk of breast cancer. Those findings were supported by an animal study at Roswell Park Cancer Institute in New York, where CLA was shown to decrease the number of precancerous lesions in early stage breast cancer, and to reduce the risk of the disease among animals.

Obesity responds to CLA, too. Studies have shown that CLA helps convert calories into lean muscle mass instead of fat deposits. Two new randomized, placebo-controlled, double-blind clinical trials from Scandinavia show that CLA has unique abilities when it comes to dealing with body fat. In one study, men with excess abdominal pounds lost an average of one inch from their waists after taking 4.2 grams of CLA daily for one month. The second study, which involved 60 obese and overweight individuals, compared body fat mass of people who took CLA for three months with body fat mass from a placebo group. Here again, the CLA group had sig-

Fight Fat with CLA
CLA has the unique ability to help convert calories into lean muscle mass instead of fat.

nificantly higher reduction in body fat than the placebo group.

Like obesity, incidence of type 2 diabetes is growing at an epidemic pace. Research shows that CLA improves several aspects of the disease. One study showed that CLA significantly lowered participant's BMI and blood triglyceride levels, two factors involved in diabetes. Although glucose levels did not drop during the eight-week study, researchers suspect that they would if the study had lasted longer. Why? In earlier tests with animals genetically predisposed to developing diabetes, CLA prevented the disease from occurring. Based on the results of this research, experts say CLA is shaping up as a powerful opponent of syndrome X, the condition made up of insulin resistance, high blood pressure, high cholesterol, and obesity.

If you do not eat lots of game or pasture-fed meat, supplements are your best source of CLA.

CHAPTER 4

OTHER GOOD FATS

The world of good fats is made up of more than fish and flax. Every time we eat, we are likely to be consuming a fat of some kind, so it makes sense to know which of the many fats that turn up at meal time are better than others. Here is a look at some of the most popular—and healthful—fats found in food.

Olive Oil Has It All

In ancient Greece, olive oil was known as "liquid gold," a name many health experts con- sider an apt description. Primarily monoun-saturated, olive oil has the ability to lower bad LDL cholesterol and raise good HDL choles-terol levels. But olive oil, which is technically classified as an omega-9, oleic acid, has other benefits, too. Here's a partial list of the good-for-you substances in olive oil:

1. Flavonoids: plant-based compounds that are powerful antioxidants;

2. Polyphenols: antioxidants with a special affinity for the immune system;

3. Tocopherols: antioxidant relatives of vitamin E; and,

4. Squalene: an immune system booster.

Three of the foremost advantages of olive oil are its availability, variety, and versatility. One of the most popular oils on the market today, olive oil is very easy to find. Olives grow all over the world, and each country produces its own special varieties of olive oil. Like wine, the different varieties of olive oil are worth sampling to find the ones you like best.

If you've ever shopped for olive oil, you may have wondered what terms on labels mean, such as "extra virgin," or "virgin." Actually, these names indicate the acid content, as defined by law. Extra virgin olive oil is the most flavorful and usually the most expensive. Nonvirgin olive oils are extracted from the olive pulp with solvents and should be avoided.

Virgin What?
"Extra virgin" olive oil is cold pressed and contains less than 1 percent acidity by law. "Virgin" olive oil can contain 3 percent acidity.

Olive oil's versatility makes it easy to add to your diet. You can, for example, simply pour a small amount on a plate and dip a bit of bread in it, instead of using margarine or butter. Olive oil is also a great addition to pasta sauces and can be used in any recipe that calls for vegetable oil, provided the cooking temperature won't be high. Cold-pressed olive oil has a fairly low smoking point—less than 300°F—so it's best for sautés, sauces, and salads, but not recommended for frying. When oils reach the point where they burn and give off smoke, they are also producing harmful free radicals.

In addition to improving heart health and lowering levels of cholesterol, olive oil protects against cancer, high blood pressure, and rheumatoid arthritis, too. As we've seen, banishing all fats from the diet is a mistake, and one we pay for with our health. Clearly, olive oil is one that deserves a prominent place in our lives. It does not have the same benefits as the omega-3s, but is a great way to cut back on overly abundant omega-6s and improve your ratio.

Fat Is Fat
Although olive oil is a good fat, it is still a fat. It contains about 120 calories per tablespoon—more than butter—and should be used in small amounts.

Controversy over Canola Oil

Like olive oil, canola oil is a monounsaturated vegetable oil, rich in omega-9 oleic acid. Canola oil contains saturated fat, too—far more than olive oil, but still less than other commonly used vegetable oils. Canola oil is derived from the rapeseed plant, a member of the mustard family. Conventional rapeseed contains erucic acid, which can lead to lesions in the heart. But the kind used for canola oil is made from genetically modified rapeseed especially developed to produce little or no erucic acid.

Canola oil and olive oil are both primarily monounsaturated fat, but while olive oil contains 7 to 8 percent poly-unsaturated fat, canola oil has 30 percent polyunsaturated, with 10 percent of that being the omega-3 ALA. Canola oil can take cooking tempera-

Canada's Contribution to Health
The canola oil sold in the United States is produced in Canada— hence the name: can, meaning Canada, and ola, for oil.

tures as high as 420°F—far higher than olive oil—and its flavor is decidedly mild, making it a perfect frying oil. As you might guess, because it has a different fatty acid profile than olive oil, it has different health benefits. Be aware, however, that some health authorities are questioning those benefits, while others feel that being genetically modified makes canola oil a poor choice, especially with so many other good fats and oils available in their natural state. Remember, too, that the canola oil often found in supermarkets may be produced with a chemical extraction process, which makes it less healthy. If you like canola oil, look for cold-pressed varieties, which are preferable.

It should be noted, though, that canola oil has shown an ability to lower blood fats known as triglycerides. A recent study in the *Journal of the American College of Nutrition* found that children and teens who had inherited a tendency to have high cholesterol benefited from canola oil in the diet. During the five-month study, the subjects consumed between 15 and 22 grams of canola oil daily, as part of a classic low-fat, low-cholesterol diet. At the end, levels of blood triglycerides had fallen by nearly 30 percent, total cholesterol dropped by 10 percent, and LDL cholesterol was 7 percent lower.

Shop Smart for Oils

Look for oils that say "unrefined" or "cold pressed" on the labels. Avoid those that have been refined or processed with heat, bleach, or chemicals.

All about Avocado Oil

Although canola oil is most often mentioned as the second-in-line to olive oil's throne, avocado oil actually bears a closer resemblance in terms of good fat content. Both olive and avocado oil are predominantly monounsaturated fats—in fact, avocado oil has more monounsaturated fat (72 percent) than olive oil (66 percent) or canola (about 58 percent). Avocado oil contains only 9 percent omega-6s, versus olive's 12 percent and canola's 10 percent. In addition, avocado oil contains a little less saturated fat than olive oil, though both are quite low.

Avocado oil has other benefits, too. It contains chlorophyll, eight of the compounds that combine to make vitamin E, an established heart-protective nutrient, plus folate and potassium, two other important substances. Phytosterols—powerful antioxidants capable of lowering LDL cholesterol without affecting HDL levels—are also plentiful in avocado oil, especially the hard-working beta-sitosterol. Some sixteen studies with humans have shown that beta-sitosterol cuts cholesterol levels and also shows promise at relieving prostate ailments, including cancer and benign prostatic hyperplasia. Finally, avocado oil tolerates the most heat of any vegetable, nut, or seed oils, with a smoking point of 520°F, making it ideal for all kinds of cooking. Avocado oil can be found in most health-food stores and in many supermarkets as well. It can also be ordered on-line.

Needless to say, the avocado fruit itself offers similar health benefits. One study found that people who ate one avocado a day for a week had a drop in total cholesterol of 17 percent. LDL cholesterol and triglyceride levels fell, too, while HDL cholesterol levels were raised. More recently, Japanese researchers found that avocado extracts were the most effective of twenty-two different types of fruit

An Avocado a Day
The 14 grams of fat in half an avocado consists of 10 grams monounsaturated fat, 2 grams polyunsaturated, and 2 grams saturated: a very healthy profile.

at protecting the liver from the ravages of the hepatitis C virus.

Say Hello to Soy Oil

The health benefits of soybeans and products made from them have been thoroughly documented. An excellent source of low-fat protein, soy has been shown to protect against various types of cancer, ease menopause symptoms, and promote heart health.

Clearly soy can be a healthy addition to the diet. But does soy *oil* have health benefits? The answer is shaping up as a "yes." Soy oil has two advantages. One, its dominant fatty acid is the omega-3 ALA, rather than the all-too-common omega-6s. Second, it has a fairly high smoking point (about 375°F), so it is ideal for baking, stir fries, and sautés. Furthermore, two recent studies from Russia show that soy oil improves cell membrane health, and its antioxidants protect fats in the body from oxidation that turns them into LDL cholesterol. These features make it a heart-healthy addition to the diet.

Remember, though, that flaxseed oil has about seven times more ALA than soy oil, while canola and walnut oil (see below) have about fifty percent more. So, soy oil's primary advantage is that it tolerates heat well, though not as well as canola. For cold sauces, salad dressings, and dips, flaxseed oil is healthier.

Meet Macadamia Nut Oil

A lesser-known contender to olive oil's throne, macadamia nut oil has a number of good things going for it. It contains, for example, a larger percentage of monounsaturated fat than either olive or canola oil. It has a high smoking point (410°F), making it ideal for all kinds of cooking and baking. Since macadamia nut oil contains high levels of natural antioxidants, including vitamins C and E, it does not produce health-damaging trans fats when heated, and has a longer shelf life than many other oils. It can be found in grocery and health-food stores, or on-line.

Macadamia nut oil also contains less omega-6s (a mere 3 percent) than do soybean (60 percent), canola (25 percent), or olive oil (8 percent), so it helps establish a more healthful balance of EFAs and is less likely to stimulate in - flammation. Another distinctive feature of mac- adamia nut oil is its omega-9 content (between 55 and 67 percent). Research indicates that omega-9 encourages the use of omega-3s in building cell membranes, making cells health- ier and stronger.

Pass the Peanut Oil Please

Peanut oil is an easy-to-find option that has a pleasing flavor and can tolerate a little more heat than olive oil, depending on how it has been proc - essed. Chemically, peanut oil is made up of about half omega-9 fatty acids, like those found in olive oil, with another third falling in the omega-6 category, and a fairly high saturated fat content, close to 20 per - cent. Because of the omega-6 and saturated fat content, peanut oil is not nearly as healthy a choice as olive or avocado oil.

Refined or Unrefined?

Unrefined peanut oil can be heated to only 320°F, but refined peanut oil tolerates temperatures up to 450°F. Unfortunately, refined oils are not as healthy as unrefined and should be avoided.

That's not to say that peanut oil doesn't have its share of benefits. Recent research at Pennsylvania State University compared the health effects of five diets with different fat profiles—olive oil, peanut oil, peanuts/peanut butter, low fat, and standard American—on a group of people with slightly elevated cholesterol levels. The results showed that the peanut oil and peanut/peanut butter diets were as effective as olive oil at lowering total and bad LDL cholesterol, without reducing beneficial HDL cholesterol. As for the low-fat diet, it did manage to lower total and LDL cholesterol, but HDL levels dropped, too, and triglycerides went up. The bottom line: while not your top choice for healthy oils, peanuts and peanut oil can make significant heart-healthy improvements.

Two other recent studies have shown that adding peanuts and peanut oil to the diet can help with weight management. Researchers at Boston's Harvard School of Public Health and Brigham and Women's Hospital found that three times as many people were able to stick to a healthy weight-loss diet with moderate fat intake, including peanuts and peanut oil, than with a conventional low-fat diet. The individuals on the moderate fat diet kept the weight off for more than eighteen months.

The Peanut Advantage
Remember beta-sitosterol, the cholesterol-lowering substance found in avocado oil? It's in peanuts and peanut oil, too.

A second study, from Purdue University, discovered that people who snacked on peanuts and peanut butter felt less hungry than when they ate low-fat snacks like rice cakes, probably because of the protein content of peanuts. Because of this reduced desire to eat, individuals who ate peanuts—even though they are high in fat and calories—did not gain weight.

Something Special about Sesame Oil

Sesame oil has more than good taste going for it. Its fat profile is similar to peanut oil—42 percent omega-9, 43 percent omega-6 LA, and 15 percent saturated fat—making it a fairly healthy choice. But sesame oil also contains antioxidants that prevent free radical formation when it's heated.

One aspect of sesame oil sets it apart, however. In the ancient Hindu practice of Ayurvedic medicine, sesame oil is highly regarded as a purifying agent for the intestines, with the ability to eliminate toxins from the body and increase life expectancy. In the Ayurvedic tradition, sesame oil's benefits can be obtained from food or by applying it externally. Because it can penetrate the skin, sesame oil is often combined with herbs and massaged into the skin, where it is said to remove toxins from fat tissues. It can also be used as a gargle to prevent bacteria that cause gum disease and sore throats.

In one study, sesame oil was shown to be effective against two types of cancer—melanoma and colon. It also is known as an anti-inflammatory and reduces bacteria on the skin's surface. Sesame oil's smoking point is below 375°F, so it is acceptable for baking, sautéing, and stir-fries.

What about Walnut Oil?

Walnut oil's chemical makeup is mostly polyunsaturated. Walnuts themselves contain more ALA than most other nuts, and walnut oil also contains these valuable omega-3s. Still, walnut oil contains roughly four times more omega-6s than omega-3s, not an ideal ratio.

Today, walnut oil is cherished for its subtle flavor. It's widely used in France, where it is a favorite for salad dressings and a good all-around cooking oil, with a smoking point of 400°F.

CHAPTER 5

UNSUNG HEROES: LESSER-KNOWN GOOD FATS

If you really want to put all the good fats to work for you, there are some less familiar varieties you should know. The names may be strange, but these fats and fat-related substances have established themselves as beneficial for a whole host of health conditions, including cardiovascular disease, liver problems, and learning disabilities.

Looking at Lecithin

Like a number of other fats, you will find lecithin in all the body's cells. Our cell membranes serve as gatekeepers, and decide which substances are allowed into a cell and which must be kept out. Those membranes are mostly made up of lecithin. This fat is also found in nerve cells, muscle tissue, and in the protective barrier around our brains. Lecithin is sometimes referred to as phosphatidylcholine—its scientific name.

Lecithin fights cardiovascular disease and hardening of the arteries, helps the liver cope with damage caused by alcohol and other toxic substances, and aids in the digestion of fats. And there have

What Makes Lecithin Special?

Lecithin is partially soluble in water, and can help transport fats, such as cholesterol, out of the body.

also been very good results from studies that looked at lecithin's ability to encourage better mental functioning and memory.

A recent review in the *Journal of the American College of Nutrition* noted that lecithin's ability to lower cholesterol had been demonstrated in several studies, including one showing an impressive 36 percent reduction in bad LDL cholesterol and a 46 percent increase in good HDL cholesterol. Similar findings were reported in a study published in *Atherosclerosis*, showing that adding soy lecithin to the American Heart Association Step 1 diet for eight weeks resulted in lower total cholesterol and LDL cholesterol in animals, without affecting HDL cholesterol.

PS Feeds the Brain

In addition to lecithin, there's another fat that's "brain friendly"—PS (short for phosphatidylserine). Like lecithin, PS is found in every cell of the body, although it is especially concentrated in the nerve cells and the brain. PS supplementation may counteract the effects of attention deficit disorder, Alzheimer's disease, memory difficulties, and depression.

For the first thirty years of life, the healthy brain is a lot like a state-of-the-art computer, effortlessly processing vast amounts of information with a network of billions of neurons and brain cells. As we age, though, brain cells die and our brains become less efficient at processing information. The result is known as age-associated memory impairment (AAMI).

Experts know that AAMI is not inevitable. We can counteract it with PS, as a recent review of scientific literature on PS, completed at the

Alzheimer's Prevention Foundation in Tucson, Arizona, concluded. PS was one of the key "brain specific nutrients" essential for enhancing brain longevity. (The others, by the way, are vitamin B complex, vitamin E, coenzyme Q10, and ginkgo biloba.)

Dozens of clinical trials from all over the world have documented the benefits of PS when it comes to improving memory and mental functions. While many of them focused on Alzheimer's patients, others have tested PS as a remedy for AAMI. As these studies have shown, PS usage results in significant improvements in memory and learning ability for individuals with and without Alzheimer's, especially those with the most serious difficulties. Recently, three animal studies showed that PS was even powerful enough to overcome the effects of amnesia-inducing drugs.

Get Cooking with Grapeseed Oil

As you've seen, some oils, like flaxseed, lose their health benefits when heated to high temperatures. And others, like olive oil, can be heated only moderately. There is, though, one oil that is remarkably healthy and tolerant of high heat, making it good for frying, baking, and even grilling, and that is grapeseed oil.

As its name suggests, grapeseed oil is extracted from grapeseeds, after they have been pressed for wine. Grapeseeds are rich in proanthocyanidins, substances believed to be one of the key reasons the Mediterranean diet is a success. The moderate amount of wine in the Mediterranean diet provides proanthocyanidins, which protect against oxidation of fat eaten during the meal, and thereby de-

Proantho-cyanidins

Highly specialized plant compounds that have outstanding anti-oxidant properties and are especially helpful for strengthening blood vessels throughout the body.

creases cardiovascular risk. Even though there are only small amounts of proanthocyanidins in grapeseed oil, this polyunsaturated oil is still perhaps your best choice for high-heat cooking. Be sure to look for cold-pressed varieties, which retain far more health benefits than those produced with chemical extraction.

Although grapeseed oil is in the linoleic acid (LA) family, with the highest LA content (75 percent) of any oil, it has a unique effect on cholesterol. As you may remember from Chapter 3, although LA has the ability to reduce cholesterol levels, it tends to drop both HDL and LDL readings, rather than only the bad LDLs. Grapeseed oil, however, has a special ability to raise HDL cholesterol while lowering LDL, perhaps because of the proanthocyanidins.

Grapeseed oil's heart-protecting properties have been demonstrated in several human studies, including one reported in the *Journal of the American College of Cardiology*. In a mere three weeks, men and women who used up to 1.5 ounces of grapeseed oil per day had increases in HDL levels of 13 percent and decreases in LDL levels of 7 percent.

But that's not the end of the story when it comes to grapeseed oil. One tablespoon supplies nearly the entire Recommended Dietary Allowance of vitamin E, a much-needed nutrient that is difficult to obtain from food sources. Grapeseed oil has another nice feature: its taste is very subtle, so it blends nicely with herbs and all types of food.

Good Fats of the Future

As our knowledge of good fats grows, so does the definition of what makes a fat good. New studies are showing that two fats long forbidden in a healthy diet—palm and coconut oil—may have real benefits.

In the Netherlands, researchers found that substituting palm oil for the usual dietary fat in the Wetern diet resulted in reduced inflammation and less hardening of the arteries in healthy men. Spanish scientists tested palm oil's ability to raise blood levels of two antioxidants—alpha-carotene and beta-carotene—in humans. Their findings showed 15 mg of palm oil per day raised alpha-carotene levels an astonishing fourteen times, while beta-carotene levels were five times higher. Furthermore, in India, researchers compared the effects of red palm oil and two other oils to see which was most effective at raising the levels of vitamin A among preschool children. Palm oil took first place.

Similar positive findings are changing the way science thinks about coconut oil, too. Once banished because of its saturated fat content, it is now being recognized as a good source of *lauric acid*, a saturated fatty acid with antiviral and antibacterial abilities. Research has shown that lauric acid can inhibit the inflammatory COX-1 and COX-2 enzymes, slow the growth of listeria, the bacteria that causes food poisoning, and kill *Candida albicans*, a common intestinal yeast that can cause assorted illnesses.

Immunity from Coconuts
Lauric acid, one of the prime ingredients in coconut oil, is also abundant in breast milk, where it is known for its role in stimulating infants' immune systems.

No doubt other good fats will be discovered in the near future. But for now, we have plenty of healthy fats to choose from—and plenty of reasons to get more good fats.

CHAPTER 6

FATS TO AVOID

Now that you know about good fats, it's time to take a look at the types of fat that fall into the other category. There are two primary culprits: saturated fat and trans fat.

Saturated Fat

The first thing you should know about saturated fat is that it is not all bad. Some experts believe that it serves a small, but important function—creating a feeling of satisfaction after eating. Saturated fat also tends to enhance flavors, and it slows digestion, so that food stays in the stomach longer. As a result, when we eat a small amount of saturated fat, we tend to feel more satisfied than after a meal without it.

Saturated fat has a big downside, though. It raises production of LDL, bad cholesterol, and has been linked to atherosclerosis, also known as hardening of the arteries, which contributes to heart disease, stroke, and related conditions.

The primary sources of saturated fat in the American diet are meat and dairy products. It is also found in coconut and palm oil, which are used in baked goods and snack foods. According to new dietary guidelines, released by the Institute of Medicine in 2002, total fat intake should constitute 20 to 35 percent of your daily calories, with no more than 8 percent coming from saturated fat—about 18 grams per day.

Atherosclerosis
Deposits of plaque on the inside of arterial walls, causing the walls to narrow and become less flexible, increasing the chance of blood clots.

Some experts believe that the saturated fat found in meat is more likely to contribute to heart disease and hardening of the arteries than dairy fat. A major European study, known as the MONICA project, compared the health of men between the ages of 35 and 64 in the south of France with those living in Ireland. Although both groups ate the same amount of fat, men in Ireland were three times more likely to have heart disease than those in France. The only significant difference in diet was that the Irish got most of their saturated fat from meat, while the French got theirs from dairy products like cheese. Until more is known about the differences between animal and dairy fat, the wisest course is to play it safe and keep saturated fat intake low. Saturated fat is listed on food labels, making it easy to determine how much you're consuming.

What about Butter?

With our nation's long war on fat winding down, experts are taking a second look at some of the most forbidden foods, and concluding that some bad reputations are undeserved. Butter is a good example. Like olive and other oils that contain beneficial substances, butter has its share of good stuff, including the mineral selenium, a potent antioxidant, vitamin A, and lecithin, that relative of the fat family with the ability to "break down" cholesterol.

But, you may be thinking, isn't butter a saturated fat, the very stuff we are supposed to keep to a minimum in our diets? The answer is yes—and no. Butter actually contains only 66 percent saturated fat. Thirty percent of butter's fat is monounsaturated, and 4 percent is polyunsaturated. As for cholesterol, a tablespoon of butter contains 33 mg, a far cry from the recommended daily limit of 300 mg. In addition, some of butter's saturated fatty acids are actually a type that does not cause blood cholesterol levels to rise significantly.

Olive Oil versus Butter

One tablespoon of butter provides 100 calories and 12 grams of fat, while olive oil is slightly richer, with 120 calories and 14 grams of fat.

So should you eat butter or not? To answer that question, let's look at a review study from France examining the role of saturated fatty acids and coronary heart disease. As the researchers point out, we've been told for decades that cutting back on saturated fats is the best way to avoid heart disease. But results from studies trying to confirm that saturated fat is the enemy have been disappointing. Only when the diet is enriched with omega-3 fatty acids are both heart disease and death from heart attacks significantly decreased.

In other words, here again, balance is the key. If you're supplementing with omega-3s, a little butter should be fine. Based on the typical 2,000-calorie-per-day diet, with a limit of 8 percent coming from saturated fat, you could have 160 calories (or 1.5 tablespoons) from butter.

Stay Away from Trans Fats

Trans fats are made up of trans fatty acids (TFAs)—good oils gone bad. They are created by subjecting liquid oil to a chemical process known as hydrogenation. When oils are hydrogenated, they become saturated fats: semisolid at room temperature and thus more stable, so they stay fresher longer. "Partial hydrogenation" means no more than 60 percent of the oil is converted to saturated fat. Hydrogenated oils make ready-made baked foods lighter and flakier, and give snacks more crunchiness than any other oil. They are also extremely unhealthy. You'll find TFAs in cookies, salad dressings, fast foods of all kinds, breakfast bars, microwave meals, peanut butter (the kind that doesn't have to be refrigerated after opening), stick margarine, semisolid vegetable oils used in baking, and plenty of ready-made snack foods.

Hydrogenation
Hydrogenation changes oils from unsaturated to saturated, making them solid and stable— and unhealthy.

Are the amounts of TFAs in these foods high enough to be worrisome? According to a recent study, the answer is yes. TFAs contribute 25 percent or more of the fat content in foods like doughnuts, pastries, crackers, prepackaged popcorn, and boxed cake mixes. Watch out for some deep-fried fast foods, too, like French fries and breaded fish or chicken patties. They scored the second highest amount of TFAs.

Unfortunately, it can be hard to tell which foods are made with TFAs, as well as how much they contain. As of this writing, TFAs are not listed on nutrition labels, although the FDA has asked that they be included starting in 2003. If you notice the words "hydrogenated" or "partially hydrogenated" in front of any kind of oil, that's a reliable sign that the food contains

TFAs. If it is one of the first few ingredients, the food probably contains a high amount of TFAs.

Another trick to identify the amount of TFAs a food contains is to add up the amounts of monounsaturated, polyunsaturated, and saturated fat on the nutrition label and subtract that number from the amount of total fat. The difference is the TFA content in the food. This only works with some products, however, because food manufacturers are required to list only saturated fat content, so unless they've gone the extra mile and included a breakdown of monounsaturated and polyunsaturated, too, you can't measure the TFAs.

Look for New Labels

The FDA has asked food manufacturers to include the TFA content of foods on new nutrition labels, which may debut as early as 2003.

The Institute of Medicine has made it clear that there is no safe level of TFA intake. Why? First, TFAs have the same downside as saturated fats, meaning they raise total blood cholesterol levels. In addition, they do further damage by elevating bad LDL cholesterol levels and lowering good HDL cholesterol in the body. And the results of the Nurses' Health Study, which surveyed 90,000 women, found that the worst fat in relation to future heart attacks was trans fat. In addition to being linked to heart disease, TFAs can also affect the way our bodies process EFAs, like omega-3s and 6s. In fact, research is showing that omega-3s are especially vulnerable to damage by TFAs.

Some experts are also concerned about other health effects that could be caused by TFAs, including cancer. Since the chemical structure of these fatty acids is essentially unnatural, no one knows how our bodies react to them or how they are processed. Remember that fatty acids are the building blocks of cell membranes and hormones, so a steady diet of these malformed substances could lead to health consequences that we can only guess at right now. To be on the safe side, consume as few TFAs as possible.

You may even be better off with butter. A recent study from Tufts University compared the effects of butter, soybean oil, and stick margarine made from a hydrogenated form of soybean oil on cellular immunity and inflammation in people with moderately elevated levels of cholesterol. None of the substances affected immunity, but there were significantly higher levels of inflammatory substances produced by the hydrogenated soybean-oil stick margarine versus either butter or soybean oil.

Don't Fall for Fake Fats

There is one other category of fat that should be avoided, although it's not really a fat at all—it's synthetic, or fake, fat. Snack foods made with synthetic fat, such as Olestra, hit the supermarkets several years ago. Food manufacturers boast that products containing fake fat help with weight loss, because the fat can't be absorbed by the body, but instead passes right through, taking with it many of the calories from foods like potato chips. If a food's list of ingredients includes Simplesse, Ultra-Freeze, Ultra-Bake, Olean, or Olestra, it is made with fake fat.

Relief from TFAs

Some soft-style margarines don't contain TFAs, and clearly say so on the container. Watch out for those that include "fake" fat substitutes, though.

How does this happen? When we eat a normal fat, digestive enzymes separate the fat into smaller pieces that can be absorbed into the blood stream. But our digestive enzymes can't break down fake fats. As a result, they stay in the digestive tract and eventually exit the body in the same form they went in, which is why we don't gain weight from fake fats.

If you read the fine print on the packages, though, you can see fake fat has several shortcomings. One, it has no nutritional value. Two, it actually robs the body of important, fat-soluble vitamins, including A, D, E, and K, which it absorbs and takes out of the body with it. Three, fake fat can cause digestive problems. Our bodies weren't designed to handle large, impervious fat molecules, so it is no wonder fake fat can cause cramping, loose stools, and other disturbances. Finally, although the packages don't mention it, fake fats are in the same category as TFAs when it comes to questions about long-term usage. No one knows what ill effects we may discover about these substances years from now. If you're trying to manage or lose weight, skip the synthetic fats *and* the snack foods. Neither one has a place in a healthy diet.

CHAPTER 7

GOOD FATS
AND PETS

Many pet owners know that fatty acids are important for healthy skin and coat in dogs and cats, but research is finding that these substances can benefit pets in other ways, too. Inflammatory conditions like arthritis, for example, can improve when pets are given the right combination of good fats. Allergies, one of the top reasons for visits to the veterinarian, can also be relieved with EFAs.

What Fats Do Pets Need?

Like us, dogs and cats can't produce some of the fatty acids they need, so they must be obtained from food or supplements. As you might imagine, however, dogs and cats have slightly different requirements. The fatty acids con-

Arachidonic Acid
Found only in animal fats, especially pork, chicken, and fish oil, this EFA is vital for good health in cats, but can increase inflammation and itching in dogs.

sidered essential for dogs are alpha-linolenic acid (ALA) and linoleic acid (LA). Both ALA (in the form of EPA and DHA) and LA are essential for cats, too, and they also must have arachidonic acid (AA). Both humans and dogs can convert LA into AA, but cats don't produce enough of the enzyme needed to make the conversion.

If an animal doesn't get these EFAs, its health is compromised, often in the same ways as humans. Pets deprived of EFAs can develop heart and circulatory problems, allergies, joint difficulties, poor coat, flaky or inflamed skin, impaired vision, slow growth, behavior problems, and damage to the liver and kidneys.

Is Your Pet Good-Fat Deficient?

One of the easiest ways to determine if your dog or cat is getting enough EFAs is to take a good, long look at her skin and coat. Dietary deficiencies often show up in the skin first. If vital nutrients aren't available, the skin can become scaly, red, or dry and flaky, with bald patches. These so-called "hot spots" are areas the pet tends to scratch or bite repeatedly. Also, the animal's coat may be dull, smell like rancid oil and even have an oily feeling. Poor wound healing is another skin-related sign of too few EFAs.

A pet lacking EFAs in its diet can also develop skin allergies to fleas, pollens, mold, and other substances. Traditional veterinary medicine treats these allergies with symptom-stopping steroids that do nothing to relieve the underlying cause of the problem and can have serious side effects. EFAs, on the other hand, improve these conditions by improving the animal's overall health, and have no side effects when given in recommended dosages. EFA supplementation takes time to work. Start EFAs when your pet has a steroid shot, so that symptoms are eased while the supplements become established in the animal's system.

Balanced Intake Is the Key

There are several ways that pets can develop EFA deficiencies. Inexpensive, generic, dry pet foods, especially those that have spent too much time on the shelf, often contain rancid fats, which are harmful to health. Also, low-calorie dry pet food is likely to be made with beef tallow, a poor source of EFAs.

Even a pet eating high-quality food can develop an imbalance in EFAs, though, because balanced intake of the omega-3s and omega-6s is just as important for animals as it is for people. In fact, according to some experts, the lack of sufficient amounts of omega-3s is the most common problem caused by processed pet foods.

This is especially true of inflammation. When a pet's diet is loaded with omega-6s, cell walls contain high levels of this substance. If the cell wall is injured, the omega-6s are released, resulting in an inflammatory reaction. Inflammation in pets can result in skin allergies, arthritic joints, kidney failure, and inflammatory bowel disease. These conditions can be treated by simply correcting the EFA balance. According to the Asso-ciation for the Prevention of Cruelty to Animals, the ideal ratio of omega-6 to omega-3 fatty acids is between 5:1 and 10:1.

Some pet food manufac-turers are now including EFAs, especially omega-3s like DHA and EPA from fish, in their products. The problem is that these oils have very short shelf-lives. Adding an antioxidant, like vitamin E, to the food protects the good fats

Flax Eliminates Pet Constipation

Add one-half teaspoon per day of freshly ground flaxseeds to your dog's diet to help her overcome constipation.

from deteriorating, but there is some debate about how effective this is. To be on the safe side, supplements are a good idea.

Considerations for Cats

Since dogs are omnivores, they do best on a diet of meat, grains, and plants, and EFAs from either plants or fish are fine. Cats, though, are strictly carnivores, and must have meat to survive. As a result, the best EFAs for cats are those from animal sources, such as fish oil.

Mother Nature designed cats to live on rodents and birds for a reason. These animals eat grass, seeds, and plants, then convert the omega-3 fatty acid ALA into EPA and DHA. When a cat eats a rodent or bird, it is getting ALA that has already been broken down. Even if your cat lives indoors and has never so much as seen a rodent, kitty is still designed to benefit from EPA and DHA from animal sources. Cats' diets should be supplemented with fish oil, which, by the way, is an excellent source of AA, the other EFA they need to get from their diet.

Since animals vary in weight far more than humans do, the dosage range for EFA supplements is wide. The best approach is to follow your veterinarian's recommendation or the suggested dosage on the product you choose. Aim for at least 2 percent of your pet's daily calories to come from essential fatty acids.

CHAPTER 8

SELECTING GOOD FATS AND SUPPLEMENTS

You want to take advantage of the benefits good fats have to offer. But where do you begin? The best place to start is by increasing your intake of the three most important good fats—the essential fatty acid ALA, plus its derivatives, DHA and EPA—and cutting back on omega-6s. We can get the good fats in three ways—from food, supplements, or by adding certain plant-based oils to our diets. There are no established Recommended Dietary Allowances for EFAs, so we have to rely on guidelines based on the hundreds of studies done with good fats.

Food or Supplements?

Certain types of fish are excellent sources of omega-3s. Among them: fresh deepwater fish like salmon, halibut, herring, sardines, tuna, anchovies and mackerel. But the amount of omega-3s in a serving of fish can vary, depending on whether the fish was raised in the wild, where it was free to eat foods rich in omega-3s, or on a commercial fish farm, where its diet was probably less healthful. In general, a four-ounce serving of wild fish should contain reasonably high levels of omega-3s, although there's no easy way to measure the exact content.

Because the omega-3 content of fish itself is unpredictable, supplements are a good way to ensure an adequate supply. Fish oil supplements generally contain 12 percent DHA and 18 percent EPA. Recommended dosage is anywhere from three to ten grams daily. Follow the dosage instructions on the product you choose.

One caution: don't assume that the infamously bad-tasting cod liver oil is the same as fish oil. It is quite different. (Its reputation was established back in the days before a mild-tasting variety in capsule form was available, and the oil had to be taken by the spoonful, not a particularly pleasant experience). True to its name, cod liver oil comes from the liver of cod and is rich in vitamins D and A. Fish oil, by contrast, supplies DHA and EPA.

Getting Your ALA

If you don't like fish, are a vegetarian, or simply want to take advantage of the distinct health benefits provided by ALA—like reduced risk of breast cancer—you'll need to get your omega-3s from plant sources, like flax, algae, or another ALA-rich oil. A typical dosage of flaxseed oil is 1–2 tablespoons per day, or the equivalent of 30–40 grams from capsules. Experts recommend starting with the lower amount and gradually working up to the larger dose. Look for organic, cold-pressed flaxseed oil, preferably in an opaque or dark container to protect it from oxygen and light.

After opening flaxseed oil, keep it refrigerated and use it quickly. Any good fat can go bad when exposed to oxygen or heat. Also, since heat destroys the omega-3s in flaxseed oil, never cook with it. Instead, use it in salad dressings, dips, and cold sauces. Flaxseed oil is safe and nontoxic in recommended doses. Larger amounts may cause stomach problems, muscle aches, and other reactions.

If you enjoy the flavor of nuts, try adding flaxseeds to your diet. They are available at health food stores. Keep them in the refrigerator until you're ready to use them, to keep the seeds fresh, and grind a small amount in a coffee grinder for each day's use.

Add one to two tablespoons of ground flaxseeds to salads, granola, yogurt, soups, and other favorite foods. Keep in mind, though, that flaxseeds are high in fiber and could increase bowel activity. This is a plus for anyone suffering from constipation, but otherwise it's best to start slow—with one teaspoon per day—and increase intake gradually. Don't forget, when increasing fiber intake it's a good idea to drink extra water to keep your digestive system operating smoothly.

Finally, if you like to garden, you might want to try the herb purslane (*Portulaca oleracea*) as a source of ALA. Widely used in Europe and other parts of the world, this little plant is a hardy annual with a succulent stem and small, thick, dark green leaves. It is a delicious addition to salads or soups and can be steamed and served as a side vegetable.

Good Weed
Purslane, an excel-lent source of ALA, should be grown in pots to keep it from taking over your garden.

Purslane has a long history of medicinal uses, and has been recommended for everything from coughs to inflammations of the eye. Today, purslane, like other dark, leafy greens, is recognized as a good source of omega-3s and vitamins A and C, and also contains calcium, iron, and phosphorus. There is no specific dosage for purslane; just use it as you would any other green and you've just increased your good fat profile.

Adding DHA and EPA to Your Diet

As with ALA, we know that these omega-3s are absolutely essential to our health, but we do not know what specific doses are required to keep our bodies functioning at their best. As a result, some health authorities say eating fatty, cold water fish, like salmon or herring, two or three times a week is sufficient. Other experts condemn fish because so much of it is tainted by pollution. Pregnant and nursing women in particular should be cautious about the high levels of mercury in some fish.

There's another consideration here, too. A great deal of the fish available in markets and restaurants today is raised on "fish farms." The diet these fish eat is vastly different from that of wild fish, who consume ALA-rich marine plants and animals. As a result, farmed fish are not as good sources of EPA and DHA as their wild cousins. If you're determined to get EPA and DHA from fish, ask the manager of your supermarket or favorite restaurant where the fish comes from.

Meet the New, Improved Egg

Look for eggs laid by chickens fed diets rich in DHA. The egg packages are clearly marked as being DHA enriched.

The generally recommended daily dose of DHA is 200–600 mg, while the EPA dosage is higher: 1–2 grams daily. You may want to choose a combination product with both DHA and EPA. In that case, 1–2 grams daily is usually the recommended amount. While studying the effects of EPA and DHA during clinical trials, researchers have used as much as ten grams per day, but there seems to be little benefit in going above five grams. Be aware that very high doses of EPA or DHA can result in a "fishy" body odor. Also be patient: it can take as long as three or four months for the benefits of fish oil to appear, especially if you're looking for better cholesterol readings.

Some experts caution that fish oil can be contaminated with the same toxins and heavy metals that are found in fish from polluted water, and advise seeking out a purified source. Another option is to choose a product derived from organically grown algae.

How Much Is Enough CLA?

Since the primary food sources of CLA are meat and dairy products, vegetarians and others who have cut back on these foods may require supplements (which, by the way, are generally made from vegetable or sunflower oil, not animal sources). Remember, too, that high levels of CLA are only found in meat and dairy products from animals allowed to graze in pastures. Given the prevalence of grain diets in today's factory farms, even people who eat red meat and full-fat dairy foods regularly are probably not getting much CLA.

Weight-loss studies have shown that 3.4 grams of CLA daily (preferably in divided doses throughout the day, or according to product directions) achieve the same results as higher doses. Therapeutic doses for humans have not been established, but research indicates that 4–6 grams or more daily may be required.

Although minor side effects, such as upset stomach, sometimes occur, these can usually be managed by taking CLA with food in divided doses throughout the day. People with diabetes or other health conditions should consult a physician before taking CLA.

Where to Get GLA

In theory, we should be getting plenty of GLA, since our bodies can make it from omega-6s. Although most of us have no shortage of omega-6s in our diets, much of what we consume comes from hydrogenated fats. Unfortunately, the hydrogenation process makes it difficult for the body to convert omega-6s to GLA, so supplements are advised.

Supplemental GLA is available primarily from three sources—evening primrose oil, borage oil, and black currant seed oil. Although evening primrose oil is the most popular, it actually has the least GLA. As a result, recommended daily doses of GLA can vary, depending on the source. Based on the GLA content of borage oil, for example, a safe dosage is 1–6 grams daily. Getting the same results from black currant oil, which contains a little less GLA, requires 2–6 grams daily. Finally, since evening primrose oil contains the least GLA, an effective daily dose is at least 2–6 grams. There have been few reported side effects with GLA, and there are no known drug interactions. But be aware that GLA supplements can take as long as six months to reach maximum benefits in the body. To be on the safe side, some experts suggest taking extra antioxidants with GLA to reduce possible free radical damage.

Rating GLA Supplements
Borage oil has the highest GLA content (17 to 25 percent), followed by black currant oil (15 to 20 percent) and evening primrose oil (7 to 10 percent).

The only flavorful oil that has a significant GLA content comes from the seeds of the hemp plant, better known as the source of marijuana. You cannot get "high" from hempseed oil, though, because it doesn't contain marijuana's active ingredient, tetrahydrocannabinol (THC). Hemp-seed oil does, however, have a healthy 1:3 ratio of omega-3s and 6s, which even flaxseed's 1:5 ratio can't beat.

Hempseed oil has other advantages, too. Its slightly nutty flavor goes nicely in salad dress-ings, and it can be used as a dip for bread, like olive oil. Cooking, though, is not recommend-ed, since at high temperatures hempseed oil forms free radicals.

Other Good Fat Supplements

If you're interested in bolstering your diet with some of the unsung heroes from Chapter 5, like lecithin and PS, here are some guidelines to help.

Lecithin is found in many foods—soybeans, egg yolks, wheat germ, brewer's yeast, apples, oranges, legumes, grains, red meat, and fish. As a supplement, it is usually derived from either soybeans or eggs (its name means "egg yolk" in Greek). It's also available as a supple-ment in capsule, liquid, granule, and soft gel form. A typical dosage of lecithin is 2 grams daily, taken in divided doses. Amounts as high as 10 grams daily have been found to be safe, and there are no known drug interactions.

PS supplements, which are derived from soybean oil, are considered safe and effective. Based on the results of nearly two dozen studies, even long-term use of PS does not appear to have negative side effects. A typical dosage is 100 mg of PS, taken three times daily.

Safety Considerations

Unless a doctor advises it, do not take good fat supplements if you are taking blood thinners, such as Coumadin (warfarin) or aspirin; if you have seizure disorders or hemophilia; if you are having surgery soon; or if you are pregnant or lactating.

Smaller Doses
If you experience stomach upset when you start taking supplements, try breaking up the daily dose into two or three smaller amounts, taken throughout the day.

There have been hundreds of studies focusing on fish oil, and the conclusion is that these supplements are very safe, even when taken for long periods of time. Fish oil can cause the level of vitamin E in the bloodstream to dip, though, so it would be wise to take a little extra vitamin E (100–200 IU daily) to counteract this effect.

A Few Last Words about Fat Supplements

Finally, if you have ever shopped for vitamins, you know that store shelves are filled with an overwhelming number of choices—and price ranges. The decision about which product to buy should not be based on price alone.

Certain factors should be kept in mind when buying supplements or oils. Otherwise, you could easily end up with an inferior product. This is especially true of the good fat sources. Since good fats have a very short shelf life, processing and packaging, for example, can make a great deal of difference in how long they stay fresh.

The best-quality supplements are from certified organic sources and should be marked with an expiration date. Look for those in opaque or dark containers, which protect them from exposure to damaging sunlight. After opening, store supplements in the refrigerator.

CONCLUSION

Getting enough good fats is a great way to keep your body in top working order. You are providing everything needed to produce healthy cells, as well as create important hormones and provide other health benefits.

As we learned earlier, our bodies have not changed nearly as much as our diet has since our oldest ancestors roamed the earth. Dietary fat was important then, and it still is today. We need it to transport fat-soluble vitamins, like A, D, and E, through our bodies. Fat makes food taste good, and it also provides a feeling of satisfaction after a meal, making between-meal snacks less likely. The key lies in decreasing the high amount of omega-6s and saturated fats in the typical American diet, and increasing the omega-3s and monounsaturated fats.

If you can make these changes, you'll gain substantial benefits—everything from healthier cells to better-looking skin and hair. In fact, getting enough good fats could help reduce your risk of everything from heart disease and stroke to depression and cancer. These are all complex conditions, and there is no guarantee that supplementing your good fat intake will make you immune. But science is now recognizing that good fats truly are good for us—and maybe you should, too.

SELECTED
REFERENCES

Albert, CM, Campos, H, Stampfer, MJ, et al. Blood levels of long-chain n-3 fatty acids and the risk of sudden death. *New England Journal of Medicine* 2002; 346:1113–18.

Belury, MA. Dietary conjugated linoleic acid in health: physiological effects and mechanisms of action. *Annual Review Nutrition* 2002; 22: 505–31.

Blankson, H, Stakkestad, JA, Fagertum, H, et al. Conjugated linoleic acid reduces body fat mass in overweight and obese humans. *Journal of Nutrition* 2000; 130:2943–48.

Curtis, CL, Rees, SG, Little, CB, et al. Pathologic indicators of degradation and inflammation in human osteoarthritic cartilage are abrogated by exposure to n-3 fatty acids. *Arthritis and Rheumatology* 2002; 46:1544–53.

DeLorgeril, M, Salen, P, Martin, JL, et al. Mediterranean diet, traditional risk factors and the rate of cardiovascular complications after myocardial infarction: final report of the Lyon Diet Heart Study. *Circulation* 1999; 16:779–85.

Ezaki, O, Takahashi, M, Shigematsu, T, et al. Long-term effects of dietary alpha-linolenic acid from perilla oil on serum fatty acids composition and on the risk factors of coronary heart disease in Japanese elderly subjects. *Journal of Nutritional Science and Vitaminology* 1999; 45:759–72.

Gylling, H, Miettinen, TA. A review of clinical trials in dietary interventions to decrease the incidence of coronary artery disease. *Current Control Trials in Cardiovascular Medicine* 2001; 2:123–28.

Han, SN, Leka, LS, Lichtenstein, AH, et al. Effect of hydrogenated and saturated, relative to polyunsaturated, fat on immune and inflammatory responses of adults with moderate hypercholesterolemia. *Journal of Lipid Research* 2002; 43:445–52.

Hu, FB, Bronner, L, Willett, WC, et al. Fish and omega-3 fatty acid intake and risk of coronary heart disease in women. *Journal of the American Medical Society* 2002; 287:1815–21.

Hu, FB, Manson, JE, Willett, WC. Types of dietary fat and risk of coronary heart disease: a critical review. *Journal of the American College of Nutrition* 2001; 20:5–19.

Ip, C, Ip, MM, Loftus, T, et al. Induction of apoptosis by conjugated linoleic acid in cultured mammary tumor cells and premalignant lesions of the rat mammary gland. *Cancer Epidemiology, Biomarkers & Prevention* 2000; 9:689–96.

Kettler, DB. Can manipulation of the ratios of essential fatty acids slow the rapid rate of postmenopausal bone loss? *Alternative Medicine Review* 2001; 6:61–77.

Klein, V, Chajes, V, Germain, E, et al. Low alpha-linolenic acid content of adipose breast tissue is associated with an increased risk of breast cancer. *European Journal of Cancer* 2000; 36: 335–40.

Nagakura, T, Matsuda, S, Shichijyo, K, et al. Dietary supplementation with fish oil rich in omega-3 polyunsaturated fatty acids in children with bronchial asthma. *European Respiratory Journal* 2000; 16:861–65.

Nestel, P, Shige, H, Pomeroy, S, et al. The n-3 fatty acids eicosapentaenoic acid and docosahexaenoic acid increase systemic arterial compliance in humans. *American Journal of Clinical Nutrition* 2002; 76:326–30.

Nicolosi, RJ, Wilson, TA, Lawton, C, et al. Dietary effects on cardiovascular disease risk factors: beyond saturated fatty acids and cholesterol. *Journal of the American College of Nutrition* 2001; 20 Suppl:421S–427S.

Nordvik, I, Myhr, KM, Nyland, H, Bjerve, KS. Effect of dietary advice and n-3 supplementation in newly diagnosed MS patients. *Acta Neurologica Scandinavica* 2000; 102:143–49.

Poppitt, SD, Keogh, GF, Mulvey, TB, et al. Lipid-lowering effects of a modified butter-fat: a controlled intervention trial in healthy men. *European Journal of Clinical Nutrition* 2002; 56:64–71.

Riserus, U, Berglund, L, Vessby, B. Conjugated linoleic acid (CLA) reduced abdominal adipose tissue in obese middle-aged men with signs of the metabolic syndrome: a randomized controlled trial. *International Journal of Obesity* 2001; 25:1129–35.

Stark, AH, Madar, Z. Olive oil as a functional food: epidemiology and nutritional approaches. *Nutrition Review* 2002; 52:70–76.

von Schacky, C, Baumann, K, Angerer, P. The effect of n-3 fatty acids on coronary atherosclerosis: results from SCIMO, an angiographic study, background and implications. *Lipids* 2001; 36 Suppl:S99–102.

Wang, H, Storlien, LH, Huang, XF. Effects of dietary fat types on body fatness, leptin, and ARC leptin receptor, NPY, and AgRP mRNA expression. *American Journal of Physiology and Endocrinology Metabolism* 2002; 282: E1352–59.

OTHER BOOKS
AND RESOURCES

Duyff, RL. *American Dietetic Association Complete Food and Nutrition Guide*, Second Edition. Hoboken, NJ: Wiley, 2002.

Simopoulous, AP, Robinson, J. *The Omega Diet.* New York: HarperCollins, 1999.

Enig, MG. *Know Your Fats: The Complete Primer for Understanding the Nutrition of Fats, Oils, and Cholesterol.* Silver Spring, MD: Bethesda Press, 2000.

GreatLife Magazine
Consumer magazine with articles on vitamins, minerals, herbs, and foods.
Available for free at many health and natural food stores.

Let's Live Magazine
Consumer magazine with emphasis on the health benefits of vitamins, minerals, and herbs.
Customer service:
1-800-676-4333
P.O. Box 74908
Los Angeles, CA 90004
Subscriptions: 12 issues per year, $19.95 in the U.S.; $31.95 outside the U.S.

Physical Magazine

Magazine oriented to body builders and other serious athletes.

Customer service:
1-800-676-4333
P.O. Box 74908
Los Angeles, CA 90004
Subscriptions: 12 issues per year, $19.95 in the U.S.; $31.95 outside the U.S.

The Nutrition Reporter™ newsletter

Monthly newsletter that summarizes recent medical research on vitamins, minerals, and herbs.

Customer service:
P.O. Box 30246
Tucson, AZ 85751-0246
e-mail: jack@thenutritionreporter.com
www.nutritionreporter.com
Subscriptions: $26 per year (12 issues) in the U.S.; $32 U.S. or $48 CNC for Canada; $38 for other countries.

International Olive Oil Council

Príncipe de Vergara 154
28002, Madrid
Spain
34-915-903-638
34-915-631-263 fax
www.internationaloliveoil.org

Flax Council of Canada
465-167 Lombard Avenue
Winnipeg, Manitoba
Canada R3B 0T6
204-982-2115
204-942-1841 fax
www.flaxcouncil.ca

INDEX

Printed in the USA
CPSIA information can be obtained
at www.ICGtesting.com
JSHW012009140824
68134JS00004B/83

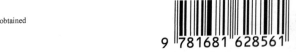